Epidemiology for Canadian Students
Workbook

Epidemiology for Canadian Students
Workbook

Kirsten Fiest, PhD

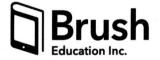

18 19 20 21 22 5 4 3 2 1

Printed and manufactured in Canada

Brush Education Inc.
www.brusheducation.ca

contact@brusheducation.ca

Cover and interior design and layout: Carol Dragich, Dragich Design.

Library and Archives Canada Cataloguing in Publication
Fiest, Kirsten, 1985-, author
Epidemiology for Canadian students workbook / Kirsten Fiest, PhD.

"This workbook was designed to provide students with an opportunity to develop skills that complement the materials contained in the textbook Epidemiology for Canadian Students, by Dr. Scott B. Patten (Brush Education Inc., 2015)."—Introduction.

Includes bibliographical references.
Supplement to: Epidemiology for Canadian students.
ISBN 978-1-55059-766-0 (softcover)
1. Epidemiology—Problems, exercises, etc. I. Title.
RA651.P38 2015 Suppl.   614.4076   C2018-900246-8

We acknowledge the support of the Government of Canada
Nous reconnaissons l'appui du gouvernement du Canada | Canada

Contents

Acknowledgements

Thank you to Dr. Scott Patten, whose years of mentorship and guidance have shaped the researcher and professor I am today.

Introduction

This workbook was designed to provide students with an opportunity to develop skills that complement the materials contained in the textbook *Epidemiology for Canadian Students*, by Dr. Scott B. Patten (Brush Education Inc., 2015).

In order to enhance skill development, this workbook contains interactive exercises that involve calculations and judgements.

This workbook focuses on 3 skills:

1) Defining and calculating common epidemiological parameters and concepts
2) Classifying epidemiological study designs
3) Critically appraising published papers employing various study designs in health research

Section 1:
A Little Math Goes a Long Way

1.1 Calculating Odds, Proportions, and Probabilities

OBJECTIVES

- Calculate an odds from a proportion.
- Calculate a proportion from an odds.
- Calculate probabilities.

Formulas you will need

$$\text{Odds} = \frac{\text{Proportion}}{1 - \text{Proportion}}$$

$$\text{Proportion} = \frac{\text{Odds}}{1 + \text{Odds}}$$

Example

The odds of getting dementia by age 80 is 0.25. What proportion does this represent?

Numerator: 0.25

Denominator: 1 + 0.25

Ratio: $0.25 / (1 + 0.25) = 0.20$

The proportion that will get dementia by age 80 is 0.20, or 20%.

QUESTION 1. The proportion (expressed as a percent) developing influenza in an unvaccinated school population is 75%. What are the odds of developing influenza?

QUESTION 2. The odds of experiencing stress during the fall semester are 1. What proportion will develop stress?

QUESTION 3. The odds of developing a rare disease during a given year are "a million to one." What proportion will develop the disease?

QUESTION 4. During their lifetime, 40% of the population will develop back pain. What are the odds that someone will develop back pain during their lifetime?

QUESTION 5. The prevalence of depression in the population over 1 year is 7%. What are the odds of developing depression during a 1-year period?

QUESTION 6. Diseases A and B develop independently of each other. The probability of developing disease A is 5% and that of developing disease B is 25%. What is the probability of developing both diseases?

QUESTION 7. Diseases A and B develop independently of each other. The probability of developing disease A is 5% and that of developing disease B is 25%. What is the probability of developing disease A or B?

1.2 Parameter Calculations

- Define common epidemiologic parameters.

- Calculate the following parameters:
  - prevalence (point, period)
  - incidence (rate, proportion, cumulative incidence)
  - odds ratio
  - risk ratio
  - incidence rate ratio
  - CIs for an odds ratio
  - changing the units on a rate

*Note: The term *disease* (or *outcome*) can refer to a conventional disease (e.g., hypertension), a health problem (e.g., obesity), a behaviour (e.g., drinking alcohol), or a positive outcome (e.g., good quality of life). *Exposure* (or *risk factor*) refers to the potential health effect of a determinant or potential determinant (e.g., cigarette smoke, asbestos exposure, stress).

Abbreviations

CI: confidence interval   OR: odds ratio   RR: risk ratio

IRR: incidence rate ratio   p: prevalence   SE: standard error

Definitions you will need

Point prevalence = proportion of a population with a disease at a point in time

Period prevalence = proportion of a population with a disease at any point in a defined time interval

Incidence proportion = proportion of an at-risk group that develops the disease in a defined risk interval

Incidence rate = instantaneous rate of change in disease status within those at risk

Cumulative incidence = incidence proportion expressed in terms of an accumulation of cases in an at-risk population specified over time intervals

Odds ratio (OR) = measure of association that divides the odds of disease in exposed participants by the odds of disease in nonexposed participants (or vice versa)

Risk ratio (RR) = measure of association that divides the risk of disease in exposed participants by the risk of disease in the nonexposed participants (or vice versa)

Incidence rate ratio (IRR) = measure of association that divides the incidence rate of disease in exposed participants by the incidence rate of disease in nonexposed participants

Tables you will need

This table is used in the formulas that follow:

		Disease status	
		D+	D-
Exposure status	E+	a	b
	E-	c	d

n = a + b + c + d

Formulas you will need

$$\text{Prevalence} = \frac{(a+c)}{(a+b+c+d)}$$

$$\text{Standard Error} = \sqrt{\frac{p \times (1-p)}{n}}$$

$$\text{Odds Ratio} = \frac{a}{b} \Big/ \frac{c}{d}$$

$$\text{Risk Ratio} = \frac{a}{a+b} \Big/ \frac{c}{c+d}$$

CONFIDENCE-INTERVAL FORMULAS:

$$\text{95\% CI Lower Limit} = \text{Estimate} - (1.96 \times SE)$$

$$\text{95\% CI Lower Limit} = \text{Estimate} + (1.96 \times SE)$$

*Note: The confidence-interval formulas, above, are for the Wald normal 95% CI approximation. CIs are not usually symmetrical.

CUMULATIVE-INCIDENCE FORMULAS:

$$\text{Cumulative Incidence}_{n \text{ years}} = 1 - \left(1 - \text{Incidence Proportion}_{\text{annual}}\right)^n$$

$$\text{Cumulative Incidence}_t = 1 - \exp^{-\text{Incidence Rate} \times t}$$

*Note: In the cumulative-incidence formulas above:
n = number of years, months, or days, depending on the time period being calculated
t = time units (years, months, or days)

QUESTION 1. Draw a line from each epidemiologic parameter to the appropriate definition.

Point prevalence

Period prevalence

Incidence proportion

Incidence rate

Prevalence ratio

Odds ratio

Risk ratio

Rate ratio

Quantifies the strength of the relationship between an exposure and the prevalence of disease

Proportion of an at-risk group that develops the disease in a defined risk interval

Measure of association based on dividing the risk of disease in the exposed by the risk of disease in the nonexposed

Measure of association based on dividing the rate of disease in the exposed by the rate of disease in the nonexposed

Proportion of a population that has a disease during a defined time interval

Instantaneous rate of change in disease status within those at risk

Proportion of a population with a disease at a point in time

Measure of association based on dividing the odds of disease in the exposed by the odds of disease in the nonexposed

QUESTION 2. The following table describes the experience of 30 people susceptible to a dangerous disease. A study of this population begins on January 1 and observation ends on December 31. At the beginning of the observation period (January 1), exposure to a contagion was assessed and coded as follows: exposed (dots), not exposed (stripes). Each month, each subject's disease status is assessed and coded as follows: free of disease (grey), ill (black), or dead (white).

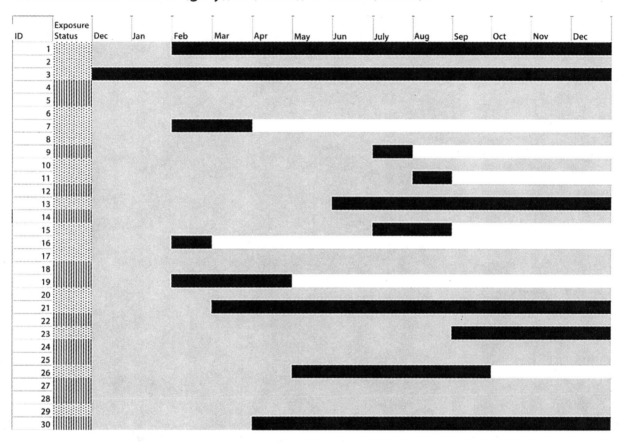

2A. What is the point prevalence of disease in June?

a) 6/30

b) 6/27

c) 12/30

d) 6/23

2B. What is the period prevalence of disease from January to December?

a) 13/23

b) 4/13

c) 13/30

d) 6/30

2C. What is the annual incidence proportion of disease?

2D. What is the 1-year (January to December) incidence rate of disease in person-months?

2E. What is the 1-year (January to December) incidence rate of disease in person-years?

2F. Using the annual incidence proportion from question 2C, what would you expect the cumulative incidence to be over a period of 10 years?

2G. Using the annual incidence rate from question 2D, what would you expect the cumulative incidence to be over a period of 5 years?

2H. What is the odds ratio of disease during the observation period?

2I. What is the 95% CI (Wald normal approximation) around the estimate obtained in question 2B?

2J. What is the risk ratio of disease during the observation period?

2K. What is the incidence rate ratio of disease during the observation period?

2L. Compare the OR and RR estimates from questions 2H and 2J. Are they similar? Explain why or why not.

1.3 Practice Calculations

OBJECTIVES

- Calculate sensitivity, specificity, positive predictive value, and negative predictive value.
- Calculate predictive values using Bayes' theorem.

Abbreviations

FN: false negative

FP: false positive

NPV: negative predictive value

PPV: positive predictive value

Se: sensitivity

Sp: specificity

TN: true negative

TP: true positive

Tables you will need

	Has the disease	Does not have the disease
Test positive	TP	FP
Test negative	FN	TN

Formulas you will need

$$\text{Sensitivity} = \frac{TP}{TP + FN}$$

$$PPV = \frac{TP}{TP + FP}$$

$$\text{Specificity} = \frac{TN}{TN + FP}$$

$$NPV = \frac{TN}{TN + FN}$$

BAYES' THEOREM:

$$PPV = \frac{Se \times \text{Prior Probability}}{\left(Se \times \text{Prior Probability}\right) + \left[\left(1 - Sp\right) \times \left(1 - \text{Prior Probability}\right)\right]}$$

$$NPV = \frac{Sp \times \left(1 - \text{Prior Probability}\right)}{\left[Sp \times \left(1 - \text{Prior Probability}\right)\right] + \left[\left(1 - Se\right) \times \left(\text{Prior Probability}\right)\right]}$$

*Note: Prior probability is the probability a person has the disease before being tested. In some studies, this is the same as prevalence or pretest probability.

Instructions

Use the following data from a sample of 169 persons with epilepsy to answer the questions below. The reference standard is clinician diagnosis of depression, and the test used is a brief depression-rating scale.

Depression-Rating Scale	Clinician Diagnosed Depression		Total
	No	Yes	
No	126	6	132
Yes	20	17	37
Total	146	23	169

QUESTION 1. What is the sensitivity of the depression-rating scale?

QUESTION 2. What is the specificity of the depression-rating scale?

QUESTION 3. What is the positive predictive value of the depression-rating scale?

a) 95.5%

c) 86.3%

b) 73.9%

d) 45.9%

QUESTION 4. What is the negative predictive value of the depression-rating scale?

a) 86.3%

c) 80.1%

b) 95.5%

d) 92.3%

QUESTION 5. The prior probability of depression is 7%. What is the PPV using Bayes' theorem?

QUESTION 6. What would happen to the NPV if the prevalence of depression was higher than the 13.6% seen in this sample?

Section 2:
Working with Foundational Critical-Appraisal Concepts

2.1 Systematic Error—Selection Bias

OBJECTIVES

- Define selection bias.
- Distinguish the concepts of systematic and random error.
- Explain selection bias in the context of common epidemiologic study designs.

QUESTION 1. Define selection bias.

QUESTION 2. Is the following statement true or false? "Selection bias can be mitigated by increasing the sample size of your study."

    TRUE   FALSE

QUESTION 3. Use the following figure to answer the questions below.

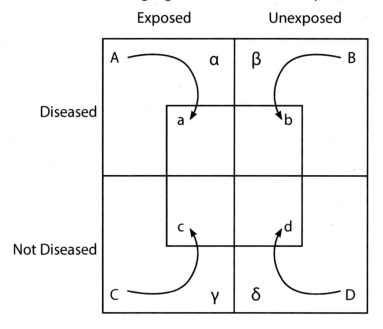

3A. Consider a prospective cohort study estimating the impact of smoking on lung cancer. To ascertain disease status, a questionnaire asks if the respondent has ever had lung cancer. If the respondent has had the disease, they are included in the study and compared to appropriate controls. Using the letters in this table, express the risk ratio relating lung cancer to smoking.

3B. People with lung cancer do not always know they have developed it. Thus, it is possible that the study design leads to underselection of people who have lung cancer. Furthermore, the authors of the study propose that smokers with lung cancer are even more unlikely to report having lung cancer than nonsmokers. If the researchers are estimating a risk ratio, comment on the selection bias that could occur from this study-design characteristic. Comment on the direction of the bias, if any.

QUESTION 4. Assume α, β, γ, δ are selection probabilities associated with a case-control study. If α and β are greater than γ and δ, will this lead to selection bias?

QUESTION 5. Assume α, β, γ, δ are selection probabilities associated with a case-control study. If α and γ are greater than β and δ, will this lead to selection bias?

2.2 Systematic Error—Misclassification Bias

OBJECTIVES

- Define misclassification bias.
- Apply the concepts of sensitivity, specificity, and predictive value to understand the effect of misclassification bias on epidemiologic estimates.

QUESTION 1. Define misclassification bias.

QUESTION 2. A major university undertook an ambitious goal: to assess the use of marijuana in the Canadian population. The university spent millions of dollars training people, equipping mobile testing units, and contacting survey participants.

2A. The study used a self-report questionnaire to determine marijuana use. Research has shown that persons who use marijuana may be unwilling to admit they use the drug for fear of repercussions. Do you think that this would affect the sensitivity or specificity of the questionnaire? Explain.

2B. Would you expect this to cause bias in studies estimating the prevalence of marijuana use in Canada? If so, what can you say about the direction of the bias?

2C. Marijuana use was also tested using urine samples and recorded in the following table from mobile testing units (which are considered a "gold standard"). Calculate the sensitivity and specificity of the mobile-unit assessments.

Test Result	Gold Standard	
	High	Normal
High	2540	600
Normal	460	23400

2D. What is the true prevalence of marijuana use? What will the mobile units say the prevalence is?

2E. If the true prevalence of marijuana use increased to 0.15 and other characteristics of the overall population stayed the same, would you expect the positive predictive value of your test to increase or decrease? Would you expect the sensitivity of your test to increase or decrease? Explain your reasoning.

2.3 Effect Modification and Confounding

- Define effect modification and confounding.
- Distinguish between effect modification and confounding.
- Describe methods to control for and assess effect modification and confounding.
- Identify the presence of effect modification and/or confounding from measures of association and statistical outputs.

QUESTION 1. Define effect modification.

QUESTION 2. Define confounding.

QUESTION 3. Complete the following diagram, adding arrowheads where appropriate. Fill in the letters *C* (confounder), *E* (exposure), and *D* (disease) in the appropriate places.

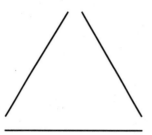

QUESTION 4. List 2 methods to assess for effect modification.

QUESTION 5. List 6 ways to control for confounding.

1.   4.

2.   5.

3.   6.

QUESTION 6. Complete the following table.

Method to control for confounding	Occurs in the design or analysis phase?
1.	
2.	
3.	
4.	
5.	
6.	

QUESTION 7. For each row in the following table of odds ratios (OR), indicate whether effect modification, confounding, or both are present.

Crude OR	OR1	OR2	Effect Modification?	Confounding?
5.00	5.00	5.02		
4.50	2.05	2.01		
4.75	2.20	7.35		
1.00	0.85	1.15		
2.96	6.21	5.99		
4.25	1.00	0.15		

QUESTION 8. From the stratified analysis output below, determine whether effect modification or confounding by the variable "modifier" is present. Which values did you use to come to this decision? Which odds ratio(s) (OR) will you report?

Modifier	Odds Ratio	Lower Limit 95% CI	Upper Limit 95% CI
No	15.75	3.33	96.63
Yes	2.59	0.66	10.45
Crude	6.61	2.49	18.22
Combined	5.36	2.21	12.96

Test of Homogeneity Chi2(1) = 3.64 P = 0.0563

QUESTION 9. From the series of 3 logistic regression analyses below, determine whether effect modification or confounding by the variable "modifier" is present and explain why. Which odds ratio(s) (OR) would you report?

Disease	Odds Ratio	Standard Error	z	P > |z|	Lower Limit 95% CI	Upper Limit 95% CI
Exposure	6.61	3.01	4.14	0.000	2.71	16.15

Disease	Odds Ratio	Standard Error	z	P > |z|	Lower Limit 95% CI	Upper Limit 95% CI
Exposure	7.02	3.25	4.21	0.000	2.84	17.39
Modifier	2.29	1.19	1.58	0.113	0.82	6.36

Disease	Odds Ratio	Standard Error	z	P > |z|	Lower Limit 95% CI	Upper Limit 95% CI
Exposure	1.34	1.23	0.32	0.747	0.23	8.06
Modifier	0.71	0.49	-0.50	0.619	0.18	2.77
Interaction	9.98	10.82	2.12	0.034	1.19	83.49

QUESTION 10. From the series of 3 logistic regression analyses below, determine whether effect modification or confounding by the variable "modifier" is present and explain why. Which odds ratio(s) (OR) would you report?

Disease	Odds Ratio	Standard Error	z	P > |z|	Lower Limit 95% CI	Upper Limit 95% CI
Exposure	6.61	3.01	4.14	0.000	2.71	16.15

Disease	Odds Ratio	Standard Error	z	P > |z|	Lower Limit 95% CI	Upper Limit 95% CI
Exposure	6.49	2.97	4.09	0.000	2.65	15.90
Modifier	0.66	0.30	−0.91	0.362	0.27	1.62

Disease	Odds Ratio	Standard Error	z	P > |z|	Lower Limit 95% CI	Upper Limit 95% CI
Exposure	5.10	3.63	2.29	0.022	1.27	20.54
Modifier	0.52	0.36	−0.93	0.352	0.13	2.06
Interaction	1.50	1.39	0.43	0.664	0.24	9.23

2.4 Random Error

OBJECTIVES

- Explain the effect of sample size on precision.
- Distinguish between components of random error.
- Describe how to increase study power.

QUESTION 1. Canada has a population of approximately 37 million individuals. In a sample of 3200 people, 725 test positive for a disease. Construct a 95% CI around this estimate and infer what it says about the population prevalence of this disease.

QUESTION 2. With a sample size of 100 000, would you expect the CI to be wider or narrower? Explain why.

QUESTION 3. We can characterize random error into type I or type II error. As the sample size increases, the risk of random error in a study decreases. What happens to the possibility of making type I and type II errors as sample size increases?

QUESTION 4. Do you agree with the following statement regarding random error? Why or why not?

"When classifying individuals included in a study into categories using an imperfect diagnostic test, we sometimes make errors in classification. For example, a test might accidentally label some individuals as positive for disease when they are not diseased. This happens randomly: that is, you cannot predict in advance which individuals will be incorrectly classified. Since this is a random process, it is random error."

QUESTION 5. Identify 3 ways to increase the power of a study.

2.5 Causal Judgement

OBJECTIVES

- Define and distinguish among common criteria to guide an assessment of causality.
- Identify the most important causal criteria.

QUESTION 1. Draw a line from each causal criterion to the appropriate statement.

Temporality	This involves random allocation of exposure in intervention studies.
Strength of association	Epidemiologic study results make sense relative to our current scientific knowledge.
Consistency	Exposure to a risk factor precedes the disease outcome.
Specificity	Higher levels of exposure lead to a greater incidence of disease.
Biological gradient	This describes whether a risk factor is associated specifically with a disease outcome or nonspecifically with many outcomes.
Biological plausibility	This is a causal inference drawn from comparison with other causal associations.
Coherence	Results in the literature report similar results.
Experimental evidence	Epidemiologic study results make sense relative to our current biological knowledge.
Analogy	Strong associations are more likely to indicate causality than weak associations.

QUESTION 2. What is the most important causal criterion?

2.6 Generalizability

- Define generalizability.
- Apply the concept of generalizability to different populations.

QUESTION 1. Define generalizability.

QUESTION 2. Can a study conducted in Canada be generalized to the United States?

QUESTION 3. Can a study conducted in Canada be generalized to Thailand?

QUESTION 4. Can a study conducted in Canada be generalized to the population where *you* live?

Section 3: Classifying Study Designs and Doing Critical Appraisal

3.1 Classifying Study Designs

• Identify common epidemiologic study designs using a standard set of questions.

Instructions

Using the following questions as a guide, identify study designs in a series of study vignettes. Identifying study design is key to critical appraisal, because study designs differ in their vulnerability to bias.

- Is the unit of analysis individuals or groups?
- Is the study observational or interventional?
- Is the directionality forwards or backwards?
- Is the timing prospective or retrospective?
- Is the intervention randomly assigned?

Use the following graphic to help you classify the study design of each study vignette.

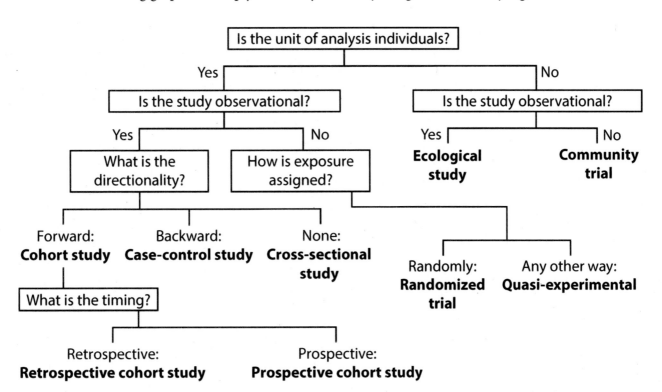

QUESTION 1. What is the study design?

The goal of the study was to determine an association between diet and the development of cataracts in an urban sample of older adults. A total of 920 people with cataracts and 920 people without cataracts were selected for the study. All participants completed a series of questionnaires, including a food-frequency questionnaire. There was a significant association between having cataracts and past dietary consumption of fruits and vegetables (odds ratio: 0.25; 95% CI: 0.11–0.65). In this sample of older adults, diet was associated with the development of cataracts.

QUESTION 2. What is the study design?

A new drug to treat nerve pain in persons with diabetes has been developed, and some people believe it may be superior to existing treatments. Investigators randomly assigned 450 patients at an outpatient pain clinic to receive either the new treatment ($n = 225$) or standard care ($n = 225$) for a period of 12 weeks. Differences in pain status (high/low) at 12 weeks follow-up relative to baseline were compared. Subjects who received the new drug reported significantly less nerve pain (hazard ratio: 0.85; 95% CI: 0.29–0.97) than those receiving the standard treatment. The new treatment of nerve pain in persons with diabetes is superior to existing treatments.

QUESTION 3. What is the study design?

Asbestos is a dangerous material. Exposure to asbestos may lead to substantial morbidity and mortality. Historical use of asbestos (per kg) and age-adjusted mortality rates associated with asbestos were examined for all countries with data ($n = 32$). Mean asbestos use from 1950 to 1959 was compared to mesothelioma deaths from 2000 to 2009. Asbestos use was associated with an increased risk of mesothelioma (adjusted $R^2 = 0.75$, $P < 0.0001$) in the 32 reporting countries. Historical asbestos use is associated with death from mesothelioma; asbestos use should be eliminated.

QUESTION 4. What is the study design?

Cigarette smoking is a risk factor for several illnesses, including some types of cancer and cardiovascular diseases. We explored whether regular cigarette smoking was associated with risk of stroke in adults older than 65. Our study had 12 132 participants (3457 regular smokers, 8675 nonsmokers) who reported several lifestyle behaviours at baseline, and who were followed for 15 years. Cigarette smoking was associated with significant increased risk of stroke (risk ratio: 4.76; 95% CI: 4.13–5.39), after controlling for several potential confounding factors, including age, sex, height, and weight. Like many other illnesses, cigarette smoking increases the risk of stroke in people older than 65.

QUESTION 5. What is the study design?

The goal of the current study was to determine if having epilepsy was associated with also having either depression or anxiety. A large health survey was conducted ($n = 43\ 922$), which asked respondents to report whether they had ever been diagnosed with epilepsy, depression, or anxiety, in addition to several other chronic health conditions. Participants with epilepsy were more likely to have both depression (odds ratio: 2.33; 95% CI: 2.13–2.53) and anxiety (odds ratio: 2.64; 95% CI: 2.46–2.82), compared to participants without epilepsy. Epilepsy is associated with both depression and anxiety, and these psychiatric conditions should be screened for in persons with epilepsy.

QUESTION 6. What is the study design?

Adverse events, such as falls and medication errors, are potential unintended complications of a hospital stay. We explored the risk of mortality (within 6 months) in patients who experienced an adverse event in hospital or within 30 days of discharge. The medical records of 75 323 patients from a large, single-payer health system were examined from 2012 to 2013. The risk of mortality was explored in individuals with any adverse event compared to those who did not experience an adverse event. Persons who experienced an adverse event were nearly 3 times as likely to die within 6 months of a hospital stay than those who did not experience an adverse event (risk ratio: 2.98; 95% CI: 2.90–3.06). Adverse events are associated with mortality in hospitalized patients. Future research should explore the effects of individual adverse events.

QUESTION 7. What is the study design?

More young people are overweight or obese than ever before. Poor diet and lack of exercise contribute to increasing obesity among youth. In this study, 26 schools in a large urban centre were randomized to eliminate vending machines selling sugary drinks and junk food, and 27 schools did not change the availability of food sold in vending machines. After 2 years of follow-up, the average weight of overweight/obese students in schools that did not have vending machines was significantly lower than the average weight of overweight/obese students in schools where vending machines were left intact (mean difference = 5.2 pounds; standard deviation = 2.1 pounds). Restricting access to vending machines appears to be an effective means of weight loss in overweight/obese youth.

3.2 An Example of a Critical Appraisal

OBJECTIVES

• Review a completed critical appraisal. (See the original study at http://cmajopen.ca/content/5/2/E386.full.pdf+html.)

Identify the stated objective.

The aim is stated in the final paragraph before methods (page E387). "We aimed to determine what individual and area-level characteristics are associated with risky driving and passenger behaviours among grade 9–12 students in Canada."

Identify the exposure and disease variables.

Exposure: individual and area-level characteristics (sex, grade, province of residence, binge-drinking behaviours, race/ethnicity, school region, socioeconomic status, and rural versus urban school location; see page E387, right column, first full paragraph)

Disease: risky driving and passenger behaviours: "(1) driving within 1 hour of drinking alcohol, (2) driving within 2 hours of using marijuana, (3) being a passenger in a vehicle driven by someone who had consumed alcohol within the previous hour, and (4) being a passenger in a vehicle driven by someone who had used marijuana in the previous 2 hours."

Classify the study design.

Unit of analysis: Includes both individual and aggregate measures

Interventional?: No

Directionality: None

Timing: None

This is a typical cross-sectional survey.

Consider selection bias.

Consideration of selection bias must be divided into the frequency estimates. There are a few points to consider. The researchers exclude children who are too young to drive from analyses concerning driving outcomes—this is probably not an issue of selection bias since this is the population that they see as being at risk, so it is probably an appropriate design decision.

Consider whether nonresponders would be more or less likely to engage in the observed behaviours. If students who drink and drive frequently do not participate in the study because they do not want to admit to these undesirable behaviours, this may lead to bias. If this were the mechanism of bias, we would expect to observe an underestimation of the effects of drinking and driving. Other important vulnerabilities to bias could arise with the individual-level response, which was imperfect (see the first paragraph of the study's results section). Only 66% of students responded, so selection bias is a possibility. The mechanism could be the same as previously discussed. The potential magnitude of the bias is quite large.

Consider misclassification bias.

Note that all exposures and behaviours were assessed by self-report. The researchers do not provide supporting evidence for the validity of their measurement strategy, so we must guess whether asking about these behaviours is likely to be accurate or, alternatively, whether it may be insensitive or nonspecific. The former would reduce and the latter increase the frequency estimates. It seems most likely that the frequency of the behaviours would be underreported (which means that the survey items are < 100% sensitive). This could occur due to fear of repercussions (were the students ensured that their confidentiality would be respected?) or because passengers might not have known when drivers were intoxicated. If this is the mechanism of bias, we would anticipate an underestimation of the association, and the magnitude of bias could be large if many students did not report the truth, which seems likely in people of this age group.

Consider effect modification/confounding.

We see little evidence that effect modification has been assessed. The traditional procedures for assessing confounding are not reported either, just 2 large regression models (Table 2 and Table 3) that simultaneously adjust for multiple variables. The best we can say is that the associations observed are not due to confounding by any of the other variables in these models.

The researchers do not discuss an apparently elevated frequency of cannabis-positive driving in the Maritimes and Saskatchewan (see Table 3).

Consider the role of chance.

The study is highly descriptive and there is a risk of type I error—with $P = 0.05$ there is a 5% chance per test and Tables 2–5 have lots of ORs.

It is worth noting that the researchers talk about what variables are greater "relative" to others and when variables are "different"—which seems to allude to statements of statistical significance that are based on interpretation of the 95% CIs. The researchers dance around issues of statistical significance in this way.

Consider the issue of causation.

As a cross-sectional study, causality cannot be determined. Indeed, this study seems to be more about identifying the frequencies and higher- versus lower-risk groups rather than trying to get at cause. For example, it would be absurd to claim that being in grade 12 "causes" risky behaviours, but it is nice to know that the frequency is higher. This raises the question of whether all of the adjustments should have been made—if you are interested in the burden, then the ORs are of less interest than the actual frequencies.

However, binge drinking could be a target of public-health-style intervention (e.g., through educational programs, etc.).

Consider the extent of generalizability.

If the results are valid, then they should be highly generalizable, since the sample is intended to be representative of the Canadian population. But generalizability should certainly be done with caution (or actually not done) to populations such as school dropouts. Perhaps it should only be generalized to youths that are in school in Canada.

Other notes:

1. Notice that the researchers use *generalization* to refer to generalization of the survey estimates to provincial populations. This is what is more commonly known as *inference*—by tradition, generalizability refers to an external population. This use of terminology is sometimes seen in the survey literature.

2. Notice that there are 2 prevalence periods (ever = lifetime prevalence, and past 30 days = a period prevalence).

3. The researchers use a bootstrap procedure for variance estimation. This is necessary because the sampling strategy involved clustering (students within schools are not independent). Bootstrap variance estimation is a way to solve this problem.

3.3 Critical Appraisal of a Cross-Sectional Study

OBJECTIVES

- Apply the concepts from the previous chapters to complete a critical appraisal of a cross-sectional study.

Using the template provided, conduct a critical appraisal of the following open-access article[1]: http://journal.cpha.ca/index.php/cjph/article/view/3838.

Identify the stated objective.

Identify the exposure and disease variables.

Classify the study design.

Consider selection bias.

Consider misclassification bias.

Consider effect modification/confounding.

Consider the role of chance.

Consider the issue of causation.

Consider the extent of generalizability.

3.4 Critical Appraisal of a Case-Control Study

OBJECTIVES

• Apply the concepts from the previous chapters to complete a critical appraisal of a case-control study.

Instructions

Using the template provided, conduct a critical appraisal of the following open-access article[2]: http://journals.plos.org/plosone/article?id=10.1371/journal.pone.0124489.

Identify the stated objective.

Identify the exposure and disease variables.

Classify the study design.

Consider selection bias.

Consider misclassification bias.

Consider effect modification/confounding.

Consider the role of chance.

Consider the issue of causation.

Consider the extent of generalizability.

3.5 Critical Appraisal of a Retrospective Cohort Study

Instructions

Using the template provided, conduct a critical appraisal of the following open-access article[3]: http://jamanetwork.com/journals/jama/fullarticle/2275444.

Identify the stated objective.

Identify the exposure and disease variables.

Classify the study design.

Consider selection bias.

Consider misclassification bias.

Consider effect modification/confounding.

Consider the role of chance.

Consider the issue of causation.

Consider the extent of generalizability.

3.6 Critical Appraisal of a Prospective Cohort Study

OBJECTIVES

• Apply the concepts from the previous chapters to complete a critical appraisal of a prospective cohort study.

Instructions

Using the template provided, conduct a critical appraisal of the following open-access article[4]: https://bmcpsychiatry.biomedcentral.com/articles/10.1186/1471-244X-12-176.

Identify the stated objective.

Identify the exposure and disease variables.

Classify the study design.

Consider selection bias.

Consider misclassification bias.

Consider effect modification/confounding.

Consider the role of chance.

Consider the issue of causation.

Consider the extent of generalizability.

3.7 Critical Appraisal of a Randomized Controlled Trial

OBJECTIVES

- Apply the concepts from the previous chapters to complete a critical appraisal of a randomized controlled trial.

Instructions

Using the template provided, conduct a critical appraisal of the following open-access article[5]: http://jamanetwork.com/journals/jama/fullarticle/195120.

Identify the stated objective.

Identify the exposure and disease variables.

Classify the study design.

Consider selection bias.

Consider misclassification bias.

Consider effect modification/confounding.

Consider the role of chance.

Consider the issue of causation.

Consider the extent of generalizability.

Appendix A.
Critical Appraisal Template

Identify the stated objective.

Identify the exposure and disease variables.

Classify the study design.

Consider selection bias.

Consider misclassification bias.

Consider effect modification/confounding.

Consider the role of chance.

Consider the issue of causation.

Consider the extent of generalizability.

Appendix B.
References for Critical-Appraisal Studies

1. Riverin B, Dewailly E, Cote S, et al. Prevalence of vitamin D insufficiency and associated factors among Canadian Cree: a cross-sectional study. Can J Public Health. 2013;104(4):e291–297.

2. Rahman F, Cotterchio M, Cleary SP, Gallinger S. Association between alcohol consumption and pancreatic cancer risk: a case-control study. PLoS One. 2015;10(4):e0124489.

3. Jain A, Marshall J, Buikema A, et al. Autism occurrence by MMR vaccine status among US children with older siblings with and without autism. JAMA. 2015; 313(15):1534–1540.

4. Thomée S, Harenstam A, Hagberg M. Computer use and stress, sleep disturbances, and symptoms of depression among young adults—a prospective cohort study. BMC Psychiatr.y 2012;12:176.

5. Rossouw JE, Anderson GL, Prentice RL, et al. Risks and benefits of estrogen plus progestin in healthy postmenopausal women: principal results from the Women's Health Initiative randomized controlled trial. JAMA. 2002;288(3):321–333.

Answers

1.1 Calculating Odds, Proportions, and Probabilities

QUESTION 1

The odds of developing influenza are 3.

$$\text{Odds} = \frac{\text{Proportion}}{1 - \text{Proportion}}$$

$$\text{Odds} = \frac{0.75}{1 - 0.75}$$

$$\text{Odds} = 3$$

QUESTION 2

The proportion that will develop stress is 0.50, or 50%.

$$\text{Proportion} = \frac{\text{Odds}}{1 + \text{Odds}}$$

$$\text{Proportion} = \frac{1}{1 + 1}$$

$$\text{Proportion} = \frac{1}{2} = 0.50$$

QUESTION 3

The proportion that will develop the disease is 0.0000000999.

$$\text{Proportion} = \frac{\text{Odds}}{1 + \text{Odds}}$$

$$\text{Proportion} = \frac{0.000001}{1 + 0.000001}$$

$$\text{Proportion} = 0.0000009999$$

QUESTION 4

The odds someone will develop back pain in their lifetime are 0.67.

$$\text{Odds} = \frac{\text{Proportion}}{1 - \text{Proportion}}$$

$$\text{Odds} = \frac{0.40}{1 - 0.40}$$

$$\text{Odds} = 0.67$$

QUESTION 5

The odds of developing depression during a 1-year period are 0.075.

$$\text{Odds} = \frac{\text{Proportion}}{1 - \text{Proportion}}$$

$$\text{Odds} = \frac{0.07}{1 - 0.07}$$

$$\text{Odds} = 0.075$$

QUESTION 6

The probability of developing both diseases is 0.02, or 2.0%.

$$\text{probability}(A \cap B) = p(A \mid B) \times p(B)$$

A and B are independent, therefore . . .
$$p(A \mid B) = p(A)$$

Then,
$$p(A \cap B) = p(A) \times p(B) = 0.1 \times 0.2 = 0.02$$

QUESTION 7

The probability of developing either disease is 0.28, or 28.0%.

$$\text{probability } (A \cup B) = p(A) + p(B) - p(A \cap B)$$

A and B are independent, therefore . . .
$$p(A \cap B) = p(A) \times p(B)$$

Then,
$$p(A \cup B) = p(A) + p(B) - [p(A) \times p(B)] = 0.1 + 0.2 - (0.1 \times 0.2) = 0.28$$

1.2 Parameter Calculations

QUESTION 1

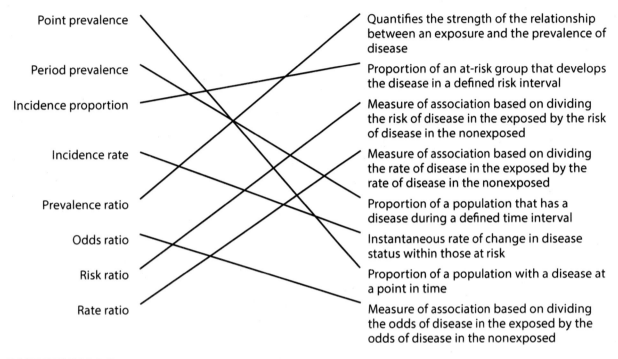

Point prevalence — Quantifies the strength of the relationship between an exposure and the prevalence of disease

Period prevalence — Proportion of an at-risk group that develops the disease in a defined risk interval

Incidence proportion — Measure of association based on dividing the risk of disease in the exposed by the risk of disease in the nonexposed

Incidence rate — Measure of association based on dividing the rate of disease in the exposed by the rate of disease in the nonexposed

Prevalence ratio — Proportion of a population that has a disease during a defined time interval

Odds ratio — Instantaneous rate of change in disease status within those at risk

Risk ratio — Proportion of a population with a disease at a point in time

Rate ratio — Measure of association based on dividing the odds of disease in the exposed by the odds of disease in the nonexposed

QUESTION 2A

(b) 6/27: a total of 6 participants have the disease and there are 27 participants in the sample in June.

QUESTION 2B

(c) 13/30: a total of 13 participants have the disease between January and December, and there are 30 participants in the sample.

QUESTION 2C

The annual incidence proportion from January to December is 0.414. A total of 12 new cases of disease develop during the year and 29 persons are at risk of developing the disease.

QUESTION 2D

The 1-year incidence rate is 12 per 249 person-months. A total of 12 new cases of disease develop during the year and there are 249 person-months of at-risk time.

QUESTION 2E

The 1-year incidence rate in person-years is 1 per 20.6 person-years. Divide both the numerator and denominator of question 2D by 12.

QUESTION 2F

The cumulative incidence of disease over 10 years would be 0.995.

$$\text{Cumulative Incidence}_{n\ years} = 1 - \left(1 - \text{Incidence Proportion}_{annual}\right)^{n}$$

$$\text{Cumulative Incidence}_{10\ years} = 1 - \left(1 - 0.414\right)^{10}$$

$$\text{Cumulative Incidence}_{10\ years} = 1 - 0.00479$$

QUESTION 2G

The cumulative incidence of disease over 5 years would be 0.214.

$$\text{Cumulative Incidence}_{t} = 1 - \exp^{\left(-\text{Incidence Rate} * t\right)}$$

$$\text{Cumulative Incidence}_{5} = 1 - \exp^{\left(-0.0482 * 5\right)}$$

$$\text{Cumulative Incidence}_{5} = 1 - 0.786$$

QUESTION 2H

The odds ratio of disease is 4.77.

		Disease status	
		D+	D-
Exposure status	E+	a	b
	E-	c	d

$$OR = \frac{\frac{10}{7}}{\frac{3}{10}} \qquad OR = 4.77$$

QUESTION 2I

The 95% CI is 0.255–0.611, or 25.5–61.1%.

$$\text{Prevalence} = \frac{(10+3)}{(10+7+3+10)} = 0.433$$

$$\text{Standard Error} = \sqrt{\frac{\left[0.433 \times (1-0.433)\right]}{30}} = 0.091$$

95% CI lower limit = $0.433 - (1.96 \times 0.091) = 0.255$

95% CI upper limit = $0.433 + (1.96 \times 0.091) = 0.611$

QUESTION 2J

The risk ratio of disease is 2.55.

$$RR = \frac{\frac{10}{10+7}}{\frac{3}{3+10}} = 2.55$$

QUESTION 2K

The incidence rate ratio is 3.27.

$$IRR = \frac{\frac{9}{119}}{\frac{3}{130}} = 3.27$$

QUESTION 2L

The OR is 4.77, while the RR is 2.55. These are quite different estimates. The disease is not rare (13/30 1-year period prevalence), therefore the OR is not a good approximation of the RR. In situations where the disease is rare, the OR will approximate the RR.

1.3 Practice Calculations

QUESTION 1

The sensitivity of the depression-rating scale is 0.739, or 73.9%.

$$\text{Sensitivity} = \frac{TP}{TP + FN}$$

$$\text{Sensitivity} = \frac{17}{17 + 6} = 0.739$$

QUESTION 2

The specificity of the depression-rating scale is 0.863, or 86.3%.

$$\text{Specificity} = \frac{TN}{TN + FP}$$

$$\text{Specificity} = \frac{126}{126 + 20} = 0.863$$

QUESTION 3

(d) 45.9%

$$PPV = \frac{TP}{TP + FP}$$

$$PPV = \frac{17}{17 + 20} = 0.459$$

QUESTION 4

(b) 95.5%

$$NPV = \frac{TN}{TN + FN}$$

$$NPV = \frac{126}{126 + 6} = 0.955$$

QUESTION 5

When the prevalence of depression is 7%, the PPV using Bayes' theorem is 0.289, or 28.9%.

$$PPV = \frac{Se \times \text{Prior Probability}}{\left(Se \times \text{Prior Probability}\right) + \left[\left(1 - Sp\right) \times \left(1 - \text{Prior Probability}\right)\right]}$$

$$PPV = \frac{0.739 \times 0.07}{\left(0.739 \times 0.07\right) + \left[\left(1 - 0.863\right) \times \left(1 - 0.07\right)\right]} = 0.289$$

QUESTION 6

If the prevalence of disease increased, you would expect the negative predictive value to decrease. You could calculate with a prevalence of 20% as an illustration:

$$NPV = \frac{Sp \times (1 - \text{Prior Probability})}{\left[Sp \times (1 - \text{Prior Probability}) \right] + \left[(1 - Se) \times (\text{Prior Probability}) \right]}$$

$$NPV = \frac{0.863 \times 1 - 0.20)}{\left[0.863 \times (1 - 0.20) \right] + \left[(1 - 0.739) \times (0.20) \right]} = 0.93$$

2.1 Systematic Error—Selection Bias

QUESTION 1

Selection bias is a form of systematic error in a study that results from defects in study design involving participation or nonparticipation.

QUESTION 2

False. Systematic errors, such as selection bias, cannot be remedied by increasing the sample size.

QUESTION 3A

Note the table here is flipped from what we typically see. In this case, the risk ratio relating lung cancer to smoking is:

$$RR = \frac{\dfrac{a}{a+c}}{\dfrac{b}{b+d}}$$

Also note the use of the lowercase letters, which indicate this is a sample.

QUESTION 3B

Based on the table, the proposed mechanism would mean that a would be underrepresented, relative to A. This would lead to an underestimate of the RR.

QUESTION 4

No, this is typical of a case-control study, where investigators select cases and controls, often choosing as many cases as possible. This would not cause selection bias, because it does not depend on exposure.

QUESTION 5

Yes, this would cause selection bias. The selection of cases and controls into the study depends on exposure status.

2.2 Systematic Error—Misclassification Bias

QUESTION 1

Systematic error in the estimate of an epidemiologic parameter that is the result of a study-design flaw involving the classification of subjects into disease and exposure groups.

QUESTION 2A

Sensitivity. The proposed mechanism would lead to an increase in the number of false negatives. The measure is unable to identify individuals who smoke marijuana as such.

QUESTION 2B

Yes, it would cause bias. It would underestimate the prevalence of marijuana use.

QUESTION 2C

The sensitivity of the mobile-unit assessments is 84.7% and the specificity is 97.5%.

$$\text{Sensitivity} = \frac{TP}{TP + FN} \qquad\qquad \text{Specificity} = \frac{TN}{TN + FP}$$

$$\text{Sensitivity} = \frac{2540}{2540 + 460} = 0.847 \qquad\qquad \text{Specificity} = \frac{23400}{23400 + 600} = 0.975$$

QUESTION 2D

The true prevalence of hypertension is 11.1%. The mobile units will say the prevalence is 11.6%.

$$\text{True Prevalence} = \frac{(2540 + 460)}{(2540 + 460 + 600 + 23400)} = 0.111$$

$$\text{Mobile Unit Prevalence} = \frac{(2540 + 600)}{(2540 + 460 + 600 + 23400)} = 0.116$$

QUESTION 2E

If the true prevalence was 15%, then the positive predictive value would also increase. The sensitivity of the test would remain the same. PPV is affected by the characteristics of the population in which it is being used (i.e., prevalence), but sensitivity is solely a test characteristic.

2.3 Effect Modification and Confounding
QUESTION 1
Variation in a measure of association between exposure and disease that differs across levels of another factor (the "modifier").

QUESTION 2
The intermixing (within a measure of association) of an effect of interest and the effect of an independent causal factor.

QUESTION 3

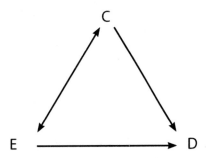

QUESTION 4
Stratification and modelling. You would compare stratum-specific estimates in a stratified analysis to determine if they are different. A *P* value from a Mantel-Haerszel test of homogeneity may be used to assess if they are different. You can also look at the CIs, though note that overlapping CIs do not mean there is no difference between the groups. Using a modelling approach, an interaction term (exposure times modifier) would be added to the model. If that term is statistically significant, then effect modification is present.

QUESTION 5
1. Stratification

2. Modelling

3. Restriction

4. Randomization

5. Standardization

6. Matching

QUESTION 6

Method to control for confounding	Occurs in the design or analysis phase?
1. Stratification	Analysis
2. Modelling	Analysis
3. Restriction	Design
4. Randomization	Design
5. Standardization	Analysis
6. Matching	Both

QUESTION 7

Crude OR	OR1	OR2	Effect Modification?	Confounding?
5.00	5.00	5.02	No	No
4.50	2.05	2.01	No	Yes
4.75	2.20	7.35	Yes	No
1.00	0.85	1.15	Yes	No
2.96	6.21	5.99	No	Yes
4.25	1.00	0.15	Yes	Yes

QUESTION 8

There is no effect modification by "modifier" present, because the Mantel-Haerszel test of homogeneity is nonsignificant ($P = 0.0563$). In addition, the 95% CIs for the "no" and "yes" groups overlap, though they are wide. Perhaps with a large sample size the difference would be significant.

Since there is no effect modification, we can move on to assess confounding. Since the crude OR (6.61) and the combined OR (5.36) are different by almost 25%, we would say there is confounding by "modifier."

Therefore, you would report the OR that adjusts for "modifier": 5.36.

QUESTION 9

There is effect modification by "modifier," as the P value of the interaction term in the final model is significant ($P = 0.034$). You would report 2 ORs, 1 for the "no" group and 1 for the "yes" group. We would need more information than what is provided in these models to do this.

We will not discuss confounding because we want to present 2 ORs here for each group of "modifier," not 1 OR adjusted for "modifier."

QUESTION 10

There is no effect modification by "modifier," since the P value of the interaction term in the final model is not significant ($P = 0.664$).

For confounding, we will compare the crude OR (6.61) with the adjusted OR (6.49). They are very similar, and thus there is no confounding by "modifier."

You would report the crude OR of 6.61.

2.4 Random Error

QUESTION 1

The 95% CI is 21.2%–24.2%. This means that 19 times out of 20, the true population prevalence of the disease will fall between 21.2% and 24.2%.

$$\text{Prevalence} = 725/3200 = 0.227$$

$$\text{Standard Error} = \sqrt{\frac{\left[p \times (1-p)\right]}{n}}$$

$$\text{Standard Error} = \sqrt{\frac{\left[0.227 \times (1-0.227)\right]}{3200}} = 0.0074$$

95% CI Lower Limit = Estimate − (1.96 × SE)

= 0.227 − (1.96 × 0.0074)

= 0.212, or 21.2%

95% CI Lower Limit = Estimate + (1.96 × SE)

= 0.227 + (1.96 × 0.0074)

= 0.242, or 24.2%

QUESTION 2

You would expect it to be narrower. The larger the sample size, the more precise an estimate will be. Since sample size (n) is in the denominator of the standard error calculation, the larger the n, the smaller the standard error.

QUESTION 3

The risk of type I error would be unchanged—this is a set value, typically 5%. The risk of type II error would go down, since it is affected by sample size.

QUESTION 4

No, random error is associated with sampling variability, not classification procedures.

QUESTION 5

You could increase the power of a study by: (1) increasing the sample size; (2) increasing the effect size; or (3) increasing the alpha level.

2.5 Causal Judgement

QUESTION 1

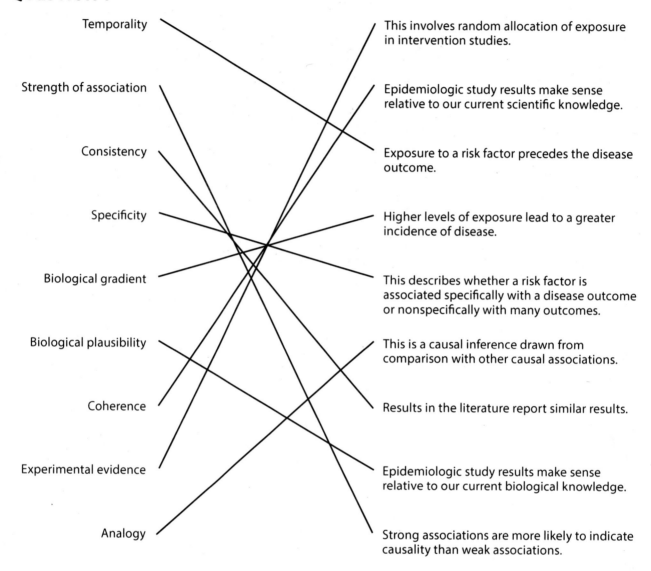

Temporality

Strength of association

Consistency

Specificity

Biological gradient

Biological plausibility

Coherence

Experimental evidence

Analogy

This involves random allocation of exposure in intervention studies.

Epidemiologic study results make sense relative to our current scientific knowledge.

Exposure to a risk factor precedes the disease outcome.

Higher levels of exposure lead to a greater incidence of disease.

This describes whether a risk factor is associated specifically with a disease outcome or nonspecifically with many outcomes.

This is a causal inference drawn from comparison with other causal associations.

Results in the literature report similar results.

Epidemiologic study results make sense relative to our current biological knowledge.

Strong associations are more likely to indicate causality than weak associations.

QUESTION 2

Temporality is commonly considered the most important causal criterion. When determining whether an exposure causes a disease, it is essential to determine that the exposure preceded the onset of disease.

2.6 Generalizability

QUESTION 1

The ability to apply unbiased estimates from an internally valid study to another population. A study must be internally valid, and its findings must not be the result of random error, to assess generalizability (which is also known as *external validity*).

QUESTION 2

Likely, though it will depend on the setting of the study, including the context of the health care system.

QUESTION 3

Less likely, as there are many differences between the 2 populations—population demography, development, and structure of the health care system.

QUESTION 4

Where do you live? Is the distribution of age, sex, health resources, disease, etc., in Canada similar in your country? If so, you may be able to generalize the results to your country.

3.1 Classifying Study Designs

QUESTION 1

Case-control study
Unit of Analysis (U): Individuals
Observational or Interventional (I): Observational
Directionality (D): Backwards
Timing (T): N/A
Randomly assigned (R): N/A

QUESTION 2

Randomized controlled trial
Unit of Analysis (U): Individuals
Observational or Interventional (I): Interventional
Directionality (D): N/A
Timing (T): N/A
Randomly assigned (R): Yes

QUESTION 3

Ecological study

Unit of Analysis (U): Groups

Observational or Interventional (I): Observational

Directionality (D): N/A

Timing (T): N/A

Randomly assigned (R): N/A

QUESTION 4

Prospective cohort study

Unit of Analysis (U): Individuals

Observational or Interventional (I): Observational

Directionality (D): Forwards

Timing (T): Prospective

Randomly assigned (R): N/A

QUESTION 5

Cross-sectional study

Unit of Analysis (U): Individuals

Observational or Interventional (I): Observational

Directionality (D): None

Timing (T): N/A

Randomly assigned (R): N/A

QUESTION 6

Retrospective cohort study

Unit of Analysis (U): Individuals

Observational or Interventional (I): Observational

Directionality (D): Forwards

Timing (T): Retrospective

Randomly assigned (R): N/A

QUESTION 7

Community trial

Unit of Analysis (U): Groups

Observational or Interventional (I): Interventional

Directionality (D): N/A

Timing (T): N/A

Randomly assigned (R): N/A